ESSENTIALS OF OPTIMAL HEALTH

By

NAWAR SABAH AJWAD

"Medicine is not only a science; it is also an art. It does not consist of compounding pills and plasters; it deals with the very processes of life, which must be understood before they may be guided"

Paracelsus

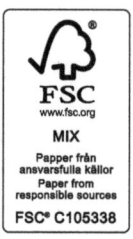

© Nawar Sabah Ajwad
Published by: BoD – Books on Demand, Stockholm,
Sweden
Printed by: BoD – Books on Demand, Norderstedt,
Germany
ISBN: 978-91-7569-696-6

Contents

Introduction

Whenever there was pain in the human lives there was always a try to decrease it. Despite that, the human pain has always been a natural process since the beginning of the evolution. Nobody wants to have pain, and nobody wants to suffer because of pain. Pain is a normal psychological mechanism that has enabled the human beings to survive during millions of years on earth. If the pain in the human physical body decreased or vanished then the chance for the human being to survive become more, simply because the pain is one of the signs of a disease process in the human body that can be lethal. Because of the existence of pain during the whole history of the humankinds, curative methods were always practiced if possible, to decrease the pain. Those curative methods have gradually developed to a huge knowledge which is known today as medicine.

We are born without previous knowledge and we acquire it with time, therefore the knowledge of health and wellness is indeed acquired with time. In the past, such knowledge or curative methods was acquired by experiences and by learning from ancestors. It was primitive regarding the ability to explain its results and the quality of the result. In the recent time, one can get such knowledge from different schools, high schools and universities in a faster and organized way.

Unfortunately, many people can not appreciate the value of their healthy bodies unless they become sick or enabled because they do not have the knowledge of how the human body functions normally and they do not know the factors that participate in the initiation of the diseases.

If we really understand the mechanism behind the normality in the function of our biological systems as one unit which is the human body, then we can understand the importance of many healthy habits and many healthy manners that enhance our health and only then we can follow those habits and manners with a high discipline. Therefore, we must answer the "why" questions regarding the healthy habits and the healthy manners that we follow in our daily life to obtain the capability to understand the importance of such manners and habits and to proceed applying them in our daily life.

The fundamental principles of the human health are based on the cause and effect principles and that means for every imbalance or symptom in the harmony of the biological systems of the human body, there is a cause. This cause can be environmental i.e. external or genetic i.e. internal. It is more difficult to deal with the genetic factors, than the environmental factors but it is very possible to decrease the tendency that genes potentially have, to establish the diseases in the human body.

When the orthodox medicine started to evolve, and its laws begun to be established during the beginning of the twenty century and especially before that period, people in every society of the world almost did not know or were particularly familiar with the benefits of the daily healthy habits and the healthy methods on the human body. Only during the last period, people over the whole world began to realize the benefits of some habits and the hazards of other habits on the health.

Unfortunately, many books that are written today about health, give the reader only the method or the habit to improve the health but they do not explain how and why these methods and habits help people to have a better health. The mechanism of action of such methods must be revealed in detail for people and in a simple way to make them believe in practicing such healthy methods and habits.

There is always a reciprocal relationship between the healthy physical human body and the healthy human psychological condition. i.e. if the human physical body become sick then the human psychological condition will be altered (for some people) with time and if the psychological condition of the individual is altered then the physical human body will be sick with time. This close reciprocal relationship will be discussed later in this book. The following chapters will discuss and explain in detail and step by step, the most effective and powerful ways to improve the human health. Through the following chapters you will explore the hidden nature of the healthy habits, their mechanism of actions and the reason that makes them essentials in your daily life.

Happiness

The happiness is a feeling that the humans usually have during happy moments of life. it is very fundamentals to realize that happiness is very essential for the normal functionality of the physical human body because there is a physiological relationship between happiness and the good health of the human body.

The environmental factors that surrounds the human body like optic, hearing and touching impulses participate in either increasing the happiness or decreasing it; depending on the quality of the impulse that is transmitted to the brain to enable us to feel the quality of impulse.

Other impulses that trigger the happiness in the human brain is internal impulses, like the memory of the humans. Who of us do not have sad or happy memories! All these sad and happy memories are saved in the human brain and whenever our senses encounter an external impulse like the smell of a good perfume that remind us about a happy incidence that happened in the past, we become joyful and glad.

The relationship between the physical human body and the feeling of happiness is very essential to have a good health. This relationship is expressed by either the absence or the presence of substances that are secreted from the brain. These substances belong to the opiates system of the brain and the spinal cord and known as endorphins and enkephalins.

Endorphins and enkephalins are morphine-like substances that are naturally secreted in the brain. Beta endorphin is one of the endorphins and it is founded in large amounts in two regions in the human brain which are known as hypothalamus and pituitary gland. If we examine these two areas of the human brain more closely we will find that the hypothalamus is a very important part for the emotional activities of the brain while the pituitary gland that is situated at the base of the brain is essential for the secretion of the hormones from every endocrine gland in the human body such as the insulin, the thyroid, the testosterone and progesterone.

Therefore, we can conclude that the happiness is a very essential factor in the healthy physical human body.

The two groups of naturally secreted opiates in the human body that are mentioned earlier, the endorphins and the enkephalins, are protein structures that are responsible for the relaxation of the body and they give a feeling of joyfulness and happiness. They are secreted in the blood stream in larger amounts especially after the contractions of the skeletal muscles of the human body during the moderate exercise at least twenty minutes. Therefore, after we have exercised for a quite long time, we usually have the feeling of relaxation, happiness and joyfulness.

Serotonin is also a substance that is secreted in the brain and have many receptors and it is considered the standard substance for the happy feelings. Therefore, those who have depression, has always a decreased level of serotonin in their brains. The orthodox medicine treats such cases of depression by giving the patient a type of anti-depressive pills that begin to give its positive effect after three to four weeks. Those anti depressive pills have usually side effects like all other medicines and the patient sometimes should change the type of anti-depressive pills several times before the patient begins to feel better.

Recently, the health care centres of many countries advice their patients to do a daily physical exercise to avoid or get rid of the symptoms of depression.

Another benefit of the happiness is that it enhances the human memory since happiness areas are situated in the brain have a well-established contact to the memory centres of the brain. Therefore, we can notice that most of the creative works of the individuals are achieved while they are happy enough since the memory of the individual and happiness enables the brain to be more creative.

The immune system of the humans becomes more potent in fighting the viruses and the bacteria that invade the human body. This is because the happy feelings normalize the secretion of many mediators, substances and cells of the immune system to the blood stream.

As mentioned earlier, the endorphins are secreted abundantly in the pituitary gland. The Pituitary gland controls the secretion of many hormones from other glands in the human body. In this way the feeling of happiness normalizes the secretion of many hormones inside the human body.

Another two classical substances that enhance the feeling of happiness are known as serotonin and norepinephrine which are secreted from specific regions in the human brain. Most of those who suffer from depression usually have decreased amount of either serotonin or norepinephrine or both.

Serotonin is secreted from a region of the brain that is known as Raphe nuclei which send signals through nerve fibres to the emotional centre of the brain which is known as the limbic system.

The limbic system is responsible for the feelings of the humans. It processes the impulses from the outside of the human body like the visual, the hearing and the smell senses to experience them as feelings.

The second classic substance of happiness is norepinephrine. Norepinephrine is secreted from a brain region which is known as locus ceruleus. Locus ceruleus is located in the brain stem of the human brain and its fibres have connections with the limbic system, the cerebral cortex and the thalamus of the human brain. Those regions have many essential and vital functions in the human brain. With out those functions the human body can not survive.

That is why the norepinephrine and serotonin systems inside the human brain are very essential, not just to enhance the feelings of happiness but also to make the whole human body functions normally as unique units that compose one complicated biological system i.e. the human body.

The physical human body can be injured or disabled at some point of time during the human life. If this injury or disability persists, it will perhaps predispose the human psychological condition to the deterioration. The suffering because of the pain that the human physical body has, is the major factor that may lead to the upset mind, irritability and uncomfortableness and even to the unhappiness and the depression. The psychological condition of the individual in its turn, has absolutely a significant effect on the human physical health.

Body Detoxification

The process of removing the toxins is called detoxification. It is a purifying process that eliminates the unwanted substances from the human body. During life, the toxins from the external environmental sources are gradually accumulated in the human body. The rate of such accumulation is various and depending upon the type of the habits of the individual. Smoking, for example, is a main bad habit that harm the human body on the molecular and cellular level. There are many examples of the toxins molecules that can be found inside and outside the cells of the human body. Carbon monoxide is one of the by-products that results from the burning of the organic materials (the substances that contains carbon molecules). Carbon monoxide can be lethal, and it is found abundantly in the smoke of cigarettes that smokers inhale while smoking. Cigarettes have more than ten thousand harmful substances that the smoker inhale while smoking. All those substances are toxins that should be eliminated from the human body by the process of detoxification that will be discussed in this chapter.

The industrialization of the societies has elevated the rate of the polluted air and the polluted water in the nature. Waste products are a huge problem in such industrialized societies. Unless the industrial countries take many procedures to minimize the toxic by-products of the factories, they will always face the problem of the pollution that for sure reflects itself on the cellular and molecular levels of the human beings and all other living creatures on earth.

The carbon dioxide that is released to the air from the manufacturing processes of the industrial factories is a major factor in the problem of pollution in the nature.

To detoxify the human body, we need an antidote that is able to bind to the toxic molecule and make it water soluble. Well, the toxic molecules are usually not soluble in water, i.e. they are not dissolved in water if they are mixed with water. We know that the water molecules constitute most of the weight of the human body and therefore the water molecules are essential in every biological process and chemical reaction that occur inside and outside the cells of the human body.

The toxified human cells are human cells that are not completely healthy and therefore, they are functioning in a suboptimal level. The degree of such suboptimality or disfunction varies and it depends upon the degree of the toxification of the human cells during life.

The process of detoxification aims to purify the toxified human cells by removing the toxic substances that are attached to the internal or the external parts of the human cells.

Those toxic substances damage the human cells structurally and functionally by impairing the normal structure and the normal composition of the parts of the cells and by doing that, the toxic substances impair the normal function of the part of the cell which they are attached to. If the toxic substances, for example, attach to the membrane that enclose the interior parts of the human cell which is known as the plasma membrane, the cell becomes less or more transportive to specific substances that are essential for the normal biological function of the cell as a building unit for the entire human body. The damage of the DNA molecules that are situated in the nucleus of the cells, for example, can cause cancer or it can cause an increased tendency to the genetic diseases.

The toxic substances attach themselves to many parts of the human cells and the only way to get rid of such toxicity is by ingesting or inhaling the antidotes that have a very high affinity to the toxic substances. Those antidotes bind themselves to the toxic substances and make them water soluble.

Once they become water soluble, they can be excreted from the human body by the kidneys through the urine or by the skin through the sweat. The kidney that is part of the renal system is the organ that filters the waste products into the urine. The toxic substances detached from their sites in the human toxified cells by binding to the antidotes and mobilize themselves to the blood stream. The toxic substances can not be released into the blood stream unless they become water soluble by the binding action of the antidotes. Once they enter the blood stream, it becomes easy to release them into urine by the kidneys. The kidneys filtrate the blood because the blood circulates continuously in the glomerulus of the kidneys. The kidneys allow only unwanted molecules and substances to pass through its selective membranes to form the urine and by this way the acidity, the osmolarity and the concentration of the blood contents will always be normal.

If the substances concentration, the osmolarity and the acidity of the blood becomes normal through the excretion of the by-products and the toxic unwanted substances, then the human cells become healthier, and vice versa.

There are many detoxifying remedies that can be found in the natural health centres. They come in the form of pills or liquids and they usually consist of a mixed of herbs that can bind to the toxic substances in the human body to make them water soluble substances and in order to release them outside the human body through urine.

Healthy Food

The dependence of the human beings on food is essential for his survival on earth. Since ancient time we eat food whenever it is possible because of the hunger instinct in us.

Before the growth of civilizations on earth, the primitive human beings haunted other weaker animals to feed on their meet. He was feeding on vegetables, fruits and seeds, red meet and sea food. The knowledge of food science did not exist at that time. The primitive human beings followed his instinct of hunger to satisfy it by eating raw food like raw food before the discovery of fire.

The human body needs a huge number of nutrients that are categorized mainly in sex categories. These categories are proteins, fats, carbohydrates, vitamins, minerals and fibres.

That classification of food is based on the type of substance that constitutes the food. Although, almost all types of foods contain a mixed of all that types of substances or some of them, i.e. we can not find a food that contains a pure carbohydrate, for example, without some vitamins and minerals associated with the carbohydrate substance of the food.

We will take every food category and we will explain its importance for the human body and for the main two processes of the metabolism which is known as anabolism (the building process) and catabolism (the decomposing process).

Protein that can be found in all types of meets is suitable for the formation of hormones, enzymes and some transmitters, etc. in the human body. The type of protein that can be found in the meets contains all the amino acids that are needed by the body to form the protein molecules. The amino acids are the building units of the protein. They bind to each other in a chain like structure to form the protein molecule.

Protein can also be found in many vegetables but there is only one difference from the protein that is found in the meets. The meets protein contains all the amino acids that the body need to form the protein molecules inside the body while the vegetable proteins contains some of the amino acids and these amino acids are not enough to build the protein molecules inside the body.

Therefore, we should eat different types of vegetables in order to get all the amino acids that the body needs to build the proteins inside the body such as enzymes, hormones and many transmitters.

The carbohydrate is essential for the body because it is the source of immediate energy. It is found in many foods such as bread, potato and seeds. The storage of carbohydrate inside the human body as a starch in liver and skeletal muscle is considered the first line of the energy storage where the energy can be released when it is needed in the human body.

The carbohydrate is also a precursor of many functional parts of the human body such as the cell membrane. When the body needs energy, the first type of food source that is utilized is the carbohydrate.

When the storage of carbohydrate in the body is partially utilized, the utilization of protein and fat inside the body begins.

The fat is essential to the human body and it is usually classified as saturated and unsaturated fat. The saturated fat is usually called the bad fat and the unsaturated fat is usually called the good fat. The difference between the two types of fats is that the saturated fat molecules have double bonds between some carbon atoms while the unsaturated fat molecule does not have any double bonds between the carbon atoms.

The ratio of saturated to unsaturated fats is approximately one to three.

The unsaturated fats are found abundantly in the fatty sea foods like salmon mackerel. These unsaturated fats are very important to the health of the human body because they are the building blocks to the cell membranes of all organs. Most of the brain cells consist of fats in their cell membranes and because of that the unsaturated fat is very important to have a well functioning brain. It has been proven that those who eat a high amount of fatty fishes every week have lower risk to have the chronic diseases of the central nervous system like Alzheimer's disease and dementia.

The unsaturated fats prevent the coagulation of the blood in the arteries and the veins. This pathological process is known as atherosclerosis and it can be lethal. Therefore, one can eat fatty fishes to prevent the blockage of the blood vessels by the accumulation of a blood component which is known as the platelets. The partial blockage of blood vessels can lead to ischemia (low blood flow) especially in the narrow arteries that nourish the heart muscle. If the blockage of the artery is completely then the damage of the tissues after the blocked artery that nourish the heart muscle is called infarction.

In this way, eating fatty fishes prevent the incidence of what is known as angina pectoris and myocardial infarction of the heart muscle.

You can buy fish oil in capsules. These capsules contain a very high amounts of the substance that is known as omega 3. Omega 3 is an unsaturated fatty acid that is found in high amount in fatty fishes. These capsules can be found in any natural health store. Take these capsules regularly during the whole life but be careful of regular high doses because very high doses of omega 3 causes bleeding in the arteries of the brain.

Omega 3 fatty acids in the fish oil can bind itself to the cell membrane of the central nervous system i.e. the brain and the spinal cord and even to the cell membrane of the peripheral nervous system i.e. all the nerves in the extremities and the trunk. This binding of omega 3 to the cell membrane of the nerve cells makes the cell membrane more flexible and facilitates the transmission of the nerve impulses through the nerve cells in the central and peripheral nervous systems. That transmission of nerve impulses is known as action potential and it is specific for the nerve cells in the human body.

Therefore, the action potential of the nerve cells becomes more intensive in amplitude while the frequency of such action potential becomes higher if the diet has enough amounts of the omega 3 molecules.

We know by fact that the normal action potentials or the normal nerve impulses are the fundamental cause for better human memory, effective learning, happiness, calmness and better sleeping quality.

Vitamins and minerals are essential for the survival of the human body.

There are two kinds of vitamins: Lipid-soluble and water-soluble vitamins. The lipid-soluble vitamins are stored in the fatty tissues of the human body and the body releases them to the blood stream whenever there is a need for them while the water-soluble vitamins can not be stored in the human body and the main source of such vitamins is by eating foods that contain them regularly.

Vitamins and minerals are important in many biochemical reactions inside and outside the cells of the human body. Vegetables and fruits are rich in vitamins and minerals; therefore, it is addviced to eat vegetables and fruits daily. Some minerals can be stored in the human body while others can not.

The most important advice in food science is to eat a balanced food i.e. to eat each of the five categories that are mentioned earlier.

Aura Clearing

The human aura is the biological fields that surround the human physical body. It consists of many intermingled layers and each layer has its characteristic features that differentiates it from other layers. These layers are very essential for the survival of the human physical body and a healthy aura reflects itself in a healthy human physical body and vice versa. The human aura evolves during the life of the human beings and its features depend on the personality and the psychological condition of the person. If the human aura is unhealthy i.e. it has darker colours and if there is a blockage between the chakras which are the links between the human physical body and the human aura, then the human physical body will be damaged and sick. This process usually takes many months and even years to appear as a disease in the human physical body.

The human aura is the finger print of the whole human being i.e. it contains every memory, thinking and emotional activity. It is like our DNA that contains our genes. Therefore, it is very important to have a healthy aura as much as we have a healthy physical human body. If we have a healthy physical human body, then we will have a healthy human aura and if we have a healthy human aura then we will have a healthy human physical body and that means that the whole healthiness of the human being is a reciprocal relationship between the human aura and the human physical body.

It is important to notice that the morphological or the pathological effects of the unhealthy human aura does not occur instantly in the human physical bod. It takes indeed a quite long time before the unhealthy human aura affects the human physical body and can appear as disease conditions according to the orthodox medicine. While the effect of the unhealthy human aura on the physical human body is not quick, we can confirm that the effect of the unhealthy physical human body or the unhealthy psychological condition can affect the human aura quickly. The reason behind such difference in the duration of time in that reciprocal relationship is due to the subtility of the human aura compared to the physical human body. Consequently, every change in the physical human body affects the human aura instantly but the change of the human aura by any factor will not change the physical human body instantly.

The change of the human aura can be positive or negative likewise the change of the physical human body can also be positive or negative.

The positive change means that the physical human body or the human aura becomes relatively healthier while the negative change means that the human aura or the physical human body becomes relatively unhealthier.

The most important fields in the human aura concerning the human health issue are the first two fields that surrounds the human physical body. The first one extends few centimetres outside the skin of the human physical body and it is called the etheric field or the etheric body. The second field of the human aura can extend many meters outside the skin of the human physical body and it is called the astral field or the astral body.

The etheric field take the form of the physical human body because it is very thin compared to the other fields of the human aura while the astral field has a very wide range and it is very dynamic in nature. The astral field is characterized by its different colours that reflect the colours of the seven chakras of the human physical body. The colours of the astral field of the human aura are relatively bright while the colours of the unhealthy human aura are relatively dark.

The sick human aura is caused by a blockage between the neighbouring chakras that prevents the natural flow of the human aura among the chakras.

The darkness of the colours is caused by many factors such as smoking, depression, pathological diseases and the bad influences of the human auras of some people. To clean the human aura and to make it healthier, we need to understand the mechanism of such cleaning in order to realize the importance of the cleaning processes.

The aim of the cleaning of the human aura is to make the astral colours brighter in order to make these colours vibrate in more harmony with each other and with the vital energy of the cosmos.

The death of the human physical body, particularly the brain, ceases the connection among the human aura, its chakras and the vital energy of the cosmos. We can notice that the awareness of the humans becomes higher when those colours are cleaned because the human aura is connected to the human nervous and the endocrine systems of the human physical body.

The opposite condition of high awareness is a state of sleepiness, senselessness and a decreased ability to memorize events. Therefore, one of the aims of the aura clearing is to enhance the human memory and to have a higher attention for the environmental events.

One of the most effective methods of the aura clearing is by using a salted water. Dissolve a halve to two litres of an ordinary food salt inside a worm water and take a bath with it for about twenty minutes but not longer. The salted water is a good medium to absorb all negative energies of the human aura i.e. the unwanted and unhealthy vibrations of the human aura. This procedure will leave the human aura clean and healthy. Repeat this procedure whenever you can. You will feel that your attention and physical energy of your body becomes better.

You can also use magnesium sulphate salt instead of food salt because it is very powerful to absorb the unhealthy vibrational energies of the human aura. You must get rid of the used water because it is saturated with negative vibrational energies and pay attention that nobody has contact with such used water because if this happens, then the negative vibrational energies in the used water will be transmitted to the healthy human aura of any one who get in touched with it.

From the beginning of the existence of life on earth, the human beings had evolved inside the salted water of the seas. By bathing in salted water, we also provide the optimal environment which had evolved our genes that we have now.

Another way to clear the human aura is by practicing meditation. Meditation is a very relaxing process that free mind, sole and the human body from undesirable energies. There are many kinds of meditations and all of them help in the clearing of the human aura and make it healthier.

Acupuncture is a traditional Chinese therapy method in the school of Chinese medicine. Acupuncture is very effective in healing because it deals with the meridians of the human body. Meridian is considered, according to the Chinese medicine, the pathways that the Chi or the vital energy from the cosmos flow through. Acupuncture clears the human aura through the therapeutic manipulation of the first field of the human aura. Acupuncture will be discussed in detail later in this book. The fire is an energy source that can also be used to clear the human aura. Shamans for example used this method since antient times. The fire from candles or any other source is a perfect method to clean the human aura because it absorbs the negative vibrational energies that can be existed in the unhealthy human aura.

Physical Exercise

Every life form on earth is characterized by the ability to move. The human being is a kind of life form like other animals. The movement of all creatures on this planet is a sign that they are alive and when they cease to move, it is an indication that they are dead.

The movement of the humans is not only a sign that they are alive, but it is also essential for their survival. For millions of years ago, the humans were primitive creature and not civilized. They haunted other animals to eat them in order to survive. To have the ability to haunt other animals means to have the ability to move. It was very important for the primitive human beings at that time to enable him to survive in the jungle.

We know by fact that the genes of the human beings during the last thousands of years are the result of millions of years of evolution of the human beings. We can conclude that the movement features of all creatures are saved in the genes of the DNA molecules and the movement or the kinetic genes inside our DNA molecules express themselves in the morphological features and the functional biology of the human beings.

Those morphological features and the functional biology of the human beings must be practiced in the daily life otherwise there will be an unbalance in the physiology of the human being.

By the kinetic, morphological and functional features of the human beings, it means the skeletal system, the muscular system, all the secreted hormones and the neurotransmitters which are evolved through millions of years.

All the living creatures move every day. It is a feature that is inherited through generations and is saved in our genes. Therefore, the movement is a natural process that is essential for the life of the human beings.

We as human beings are the result of our external environment and the genes are one of the fundamental elements of the environment. Every atom, cell, tissue, organ in the human body is in constant movement and we should maintain such movement in order to be alive. The purpose of the physical exercise is to contract the skeletal muscles that are attached to the skeleton. These muscles are voluntary muscles i.e. we have control over their contraction. The physical exercise aims also to contract involuntary muscles like the heart and the diaphragm. They are called involuntary muscles because we do not have a direct control over their contractions. The physical exercise like walking and running are very important to have a better physiological condition. Physiology is the science that deals with the normal functions of the organs and systems of the human body. The physical exercise lowers the heart rate. It is always better to have a lower normal heart rate. During the physical exercise the heart muscle pumps the blood to the aorta artery which is the first and biggest artery that rises from the heart. The aorta artery distributes the blood to the whole body through smaller arteries. The heart is an involuntary muscle that participates in having a better physiological condition. When we exercise, we contract the skeletal muscle in order to move the body. This contraction of the skeletal muscles need energy in the form of glucose molecule. Glucose molecules are released from the starch that is saved in the liver and inside the skeletal muscle. This means that the skeletal muscle needs more glucose molecules as a fuel to be contracted harder and at an increased rate during the physical exercise. The only way that can transfer higher concentration of the glucose molecules to the skeletal muscle is by circulating more blood through the skeletal muscle. The blood circulation in the tissues of the human body depends upon the heart pumping rate. When the rate of the heart beat increases, the blood circulation in the tissues increases also and vice versa.

The increased circulation of the blood in the brain regions provides more blood flow to the small capillaries of the brain and subsequently, the blood provides more oxygen to the nerve cells and more nutrients in the form of glucose molecules to the brain nerve cells. At the same time, the blood that leaves the capillaries of the brain takes the waste products in the form of carbon dioxide to the lungs where they exhaled outside the human body.

In this way, the brain nerve cells are nourished with oxygen and get rid of the waste products effectively. Subsequently, the brain nerve cells become healthier and more efficient in transmitting nerve impulses.

By the same mechanism, every cell in the different tissues of the human body works efficiently. When we examine the lungs and the brain tissues after the physical exercise, we can notice that the lung capacity is increased and the branching of the small capillaries in the lungs has increased too. The same thing occurs to the brain different regions. If the brain different regions work optimally, then we can conclude that the endocrine system and the whole endocrine system works normally because the central nervous of the brain and the spinal cord connects to the whole endocrine system by the pituitary gland which is situated at the base of the brain and secrets many hormones to control the function of other endocrine glands such as the thyroid, the adrenal, the testicle glands.

The endocrine glands secret many hormones into the blood stream. The hormones are biological molecules that are carried by the blood to almost every cell of the human body. These hormones bind to their receptors on the surfaces of the membranes of the human cells and cause remarkable changes in those cells. Those changes appear in the tissues and the organs of the human body later. The excessive secretion of some hormones can cause damage to the tissues of the organs but all the secretion of hormones during and after the physical exercise is optimized, balanced and beneficial for the human body.

If the person continues to do physical exercises then, the heart muscle like every muscle in the human body becomes stronger with time. After a few months of regular physical exercise and when the body is relaxed i.e. without any physical exercise, it pumps more blood in each beat which means that the blood flow to the tissues of the human body becomes higher. That is because the size of the heart muscle has become larger and therefore, the outflow of the blood in each beat becomes larger. But what about the heart rate? The heart rate is defined as the number of the heart beats per one minute and it becomes lower when the person does a physical exercise regularly.

The athletics that runs a marathon has always a low heart rate and a high pumped amount of blood in each heartbeat. Therefore, when they run a marathon, the heart can supply the whole body with the oxygenated blood when the heart rate becomes higher.

While the athletics have low heart rates, the passive people who do not exercise regularly usually have a higher heart rate when they are relaxed and when they do a physical exercise like running or jogging, the heart rate must become higher to ensure a sufficient amount of blood to the whole human body. But the passive individuals have already a high heart rate and therefore, the heart rate becomes very high during the exercise time which is not appropriate for the normal function of the heart muscle.

The physical exercise enhances the psychological endurance and increase the stress resistance. That is because after each physical exercise period, the cortisol hormone which is released in stress situations from the adrenal glands, becomes less in the blood stream. Beside that, the biological endorphins are secreted from the bran which calm down the individual and give a feeling of happiness and relaxation.

The physical exercise strengthens the skeleton because during each contraction of a skeletal muscle, there is a force that treys to move the bones of the joint. The muscles are inserted in the bones by the tendons. If that force which is applied by the skeletal (striated) muscles continue, a group of cells inside the bone tissue begin to build up the calcified bone tissues. These cells are called osteoblasts. While the osteoblast builds up the bone and increase its density, the opposite occurs by a group of cells that shrink the bone tissue and decrease its density. These cells are called the osteoclasts. The exercise is not enough to have a solid and strong skeleton. There must be food that are eaten by the individual to build up the skeleton. The most important food is the milk because the milk contains the calcium that is needed as building blocks for the bone tissues and the milk contains also vitamin D which works as a cofactor to start the biological reaction that are needed to build up the bone tissues. Vitamin D is found in many foods such as sea foods and the human body can obtains it from the ultra violet rays that is found in the sun light.

But at which time during the day should we do the physical exercise? To answer this question, we should learn little about the biochemistry of the protein, the fats and the carbohydrates inside the human body. Well, if the individual started to jog or run on an empty stomach in the morning for example, then the energy that the skeletal muscles need during the physical exercise originate from the protein that the skeletal muscle is made of and from the fats of the adipose tissue (the fatty tissue). It is good to lose some weight through the burning of the adipose tissue, but it is not good to lose the protein that the skeletal muscle is made of.

What about if the individual does the physical exercise directly after the meal? Well, in this case the energy that is needed by the skeletal muscle in order to contracts is originated from the food the individual has just eaten and if the individual wants to consume some calories from fatty tissues, then it will not be possible. Therefore, the best time to do the physical exercise is about three to four hours after we have eaten the meal. Most of the people who exercise prefer the time after their daily job has finished. In this way, they get rid of the stress of the day and they can consume calories from the adipose tissue too.

But how long time do we need to get some benefit from the physical exercise? Concerning the loss of weight, it is recommended to jog or run not less than twenty minutes because during the first minutes of jogging, the carbohydrates and little protein of the skeletal muscles begins to mobilize and are used as fuel for the contraction of the skeletal muscles. After about twenty minutes, the fatty tissues begin to be mobilized and it is used as fuel for the contraction of the skeletal muscle that are active during the physical exercise.

When you need to increase your physical and psychological conditions, it is recommended to jog or run for any period.

It has been proved that the physical exercise has a numerous positive effect on the brain. Physical exercise decreases the reaction time. Reaction time is the time we need to respond to anything that occurs in our environment. Only one time of physical exercise gives a better sleep during the night. It also decreases the symptoms of the depression. In addition of that, the physical exercise enhances the memory, the attention and the learning abilities. All this positive effect on the brain occurs due to the increased numbers of the new nerve cells because of the increased blood circulation to the small brain arterioles that nourish the brain tissues. The physical exercise decreases the level of cortisol and adrenalin in the blood. This make the person calmer and the person do not respond easily to the stressful situations. The explanation for that can be the high blood flow through every tissue in the human body inclusive the tissues of the pituitary gland (the major gland in the human body) which controls the secretion of other glands in the human body inclusive the adrenal glands (suprarenal glands) which secrets the cortisol and the adrenalin hormones to the blood stream. These hormones are responsible for the stress feelings and the low stress threshold in many persons. The feed back impulses by the same hormones in the blood stream can stop more secretion of the stress hormones (cortisol and adrenalin) into the blood stream.

Regular physical exercise increases the sensibility of all cells to the insulin. The cells need insulin to transport the glucose molecules into the interior side of the cells in order to use the glucose molecules as a source of energy to ensure the normal function of the cells and tissues. Regular physical exercise also normalizes the blood values such as cholesterol which lead to low tendency of atherosclerosis of the blood vessels especially in the narrow arteries that nourish the heart muscle which minimize the risk for the heart infarct. The blood pressure decreases after each physical exercise and the blood flow to the skeletal muscles and the heart increases.

The Immune System

The human body has lived in our natural environment for millions of years. This environment has had a hostile character because there are a huge number of microbes, parasites and other microorganisms that were lethal to the human beings.

The process of starting and establishing the disease inside the human body is called the pathogenesis and the microbes or the parasite that cause the pathogenesis is known as the pathogen such as the bacteria and viruses. From the evolutionary point of view, the immune system of the human body has been adapted to the environmental threats such as bacteria, viruses and parasites through millions of years. Consequently, the human body can identify the invading microbes inside the human body, and it has the ability to fight these microbes by producing many immune cells which can attack and eliminate the potential danger of the microbes and the parasites. The mechanism of the immune system is very specific for billions of microbes and foreign substances. This particular type of the human immune system is called the adaptive immunity and it is mediated mainly by cells which are known as B sells (humoral immunity) and by T cells (cell mediated immunity). The T cells are an excellent fighter against viruses while B cells are excellent fighter against bacteria. The other type of the human immune system is called the innate immunity and its response to the pathogens is immediate while the response of the adaptive immune system is not immediate and can take several days in order to begin fighting the microbes and eliminate them.

There are many pathogens but those who are very small in size like bacteria and viruses are called microbes.

To enhance the immune system is one of the ways that is very powerful to prevent the diseases inside the human body. To enhance the immune system means to make the immune cells more active and powerful, to increase their numbers and to increase the speed in which they can target the pathogens and destroy them quickly.

There are many methods to increase those abilities of the immune system and one of them is by eating a balanced food, especially food that contain chemical substances that enhance the efficiency of the immune system on the cellular level.

The innate immune system that defends the human body against microbes and foreign bodies by attacking and engulfing many types of pathogens has an immediate response compared to the adaptive immune system which delays few days before its response become efficient.

The cells of the innate immune system include those which are found the lining interior layer of respiratory, digestive, urinary and sexual organs. Those lining layers are called the epithelial layers and they are the first barrier against external microbes that may try to transport themselves into the blood stream through those epithelial layers. The immune cells that are found in those layers are of several types such as the macrophages, the neutrophils and the natural killer cells (NK).

Those cells are considered the first line of defence against the microbes and the foreign bodies and they belong to the innate immune system.

If we want to enhance the innate immune system against any potential threats of the microbes and foreign bodies, then we should enhance those immune cells by enhancing their functions and the efficiency of their work inside the human body. That can be achieved by providing the human body with the nutrients that potentiate the function of those immune cells. The most important nutrients to enhance the innate immune system are the antioxidants.

The antioxidant are the substances that can be found naturally in all vegetables and fruits in various amounts depending on the type of the vegetable or the fruit. The antioxidants fight other substances in the human body that damage the human cells which are known as the free radicles. The antioxidants in the vegetables and the fruits are reducing the oxidative effect of the free radicles on the cells of the human body and by doing that the antioxidants prevent all the cells of the human body from being oxidized and damaged.

The antioxidants that are found in the raw garlic are very optimizing for the function of T cells (cell mediated immunity) and B cells (humoral immunity) and the cells of the innate immune system. Garlic contains dozens of antioxidants that are very powerful in enhancing the whole immune system especially the T cells that participate in the process of weakening and eliminating the viruses that invade the human body. B cells are responsible for the producing of antibodies which are very important in eliminating the bacteria from the infected tissues. B cells surrounds the pathogens and make the easily engulphed by specialized immune cells which are known as the macrophages and the natural killer cells (NK).

You can get garlic in the form of pills or tablets that are found under many labels in the natural health centres. Agent garlic extract is the most odourless form and it enhances all the types of the immune system especially the cell mediated immunity.

To enhance the immune system of the human body has a major benefit which is to prevent the infectious diseases to be established inside the human body. But be careful not to take high doses of garlic extracts under long time because high dosage during a long period of time can stimulates the immune system extremely and that can cause auto immune diseases i.e. the human immune cells begin to identify the natural cells of the human body as foreign bodies and attack them which can damage the tissues.

There is only one disadvantage of enhancing the immune system under long period of time. We know that the repeated infections inside the human body enhances the adaptive immune system (the humoral and the cell mediated immunity). That repeated exposure to the different pathogens stimulate specialized cells which are known as the memory cells which make the response of the immune system when it encounters the same pathogen more aggressive and quicker. If we use a protective method like garlic tablets, then we do not be infected easily but we lose the stimulation of the memory cells during the process of infection which make the immune system more efficient in battling the pathogens and the microbes.

Another substance that enhance the immune system of the human body is the vitamin C. Vitamin C stimulate all the reactions of the adaptive and innate immune cells. Therefore, it is recommended to take garlic tablets together with vitamin C in the natural form or in the tablets form during influenza for example. Vitamin C is very safe i.e. it is not toxic even in very high doses. In fact, it is very detoxifying for the colon if we take it in high doses on an empty stomach in the morning.

The immune system functions optimally during the rest period. Therefore, we should get as much rest as possible during the period of any disease because the human immune system functions optimally and efficiently during the relaxation. The stress of any kind can increase the cortisol level in the blood and cortisol is an anti-inflammatory substance which means that the inflammatory process will be decreased in the human body. We know by fact that the inflammatory process is a natural and an essential process in the eliminating of the microbes that invade the human body and that is why we need to relax and do not be exposed to any physical or psychological stress during the period of illness.

Litheness and Obesity

Obesity is considered one of the recent problems of the modern societies. The modern societies are characterized by little physical movement of its individuals due to the presence of the facilities that can transport people such as the cars, the airplanes, the motorcycles etc.

Too many hours of sitting in front of the computers is also a sign of the passivity of the modern societies. All these factors have participated in the decreased physical movement of the people which made the individuals depend on those facilities instead of depending upon themselves in doing the daily tasks.

Consequently, the individuals in the modern societies do not utilize the daily ingested food in the metabolism which produces the energy that the cells of the human body need. Instead, the individual, because of the absence of the physical movement, saves the ingested food as fats molecules in the fatty tissue which is known as the adipose tissue inside the human body.

The high calories food like the animal fats is another factor in the obesity. If we eat food that contains calories more than calories which we need daily, the extra calories will be saved as adipose tissue (fatty tissue) inside the human body.

The classical and biological region in which the adipose tissue accumulates abundantly inside the female body is the hips region while the classical and biological region of the human body where the adipose tissue accumulate abundantly is the abdomen region (around the stomach and beneath the skin of the abdominal region).

The fact of the input of calories as food must be equal to the output of calories which transform to the energy that is needed by the human body is fundamental in the steadiness of the human body's weight during the time i.e. the human body will not lose or gain any weight in the form of adipose tissue.

A lithe person has a very little amount of the adipose tissue in the body. This is very important in the working of the heart muscle. Those who are obese have higher heart rate in relaxed conditions because the heart muscle must pump the blood to a larger mass of tissues of the human body since the fatty or the adipose tissue is part of the tissues of the human body and the blood should circulate through it in order to make it alive like other tissues inside the human body that need blood to continue being alive. Therefore, we can notice and conclude that the lithe person needs little blood to nourishing all the tissues of the human body and therefore, the heart muscle need fewer contractions per minute (the heart rate) in order to nourish all the tissues of the human body including the adipose tissue.

We can also conclude that the adipose tissue in obese people does not have a huge roll in the healthiness of the human body and the human body has a disadvantage if it accumulates such adipose tissue. The only beneficial feature of the adipose tissue is that it provides the human body with energy through the catabolism (the process of breaking down the macromolecules into simpler forms) of such adipose tissue. The second beneficial feature of the adipose tissue is that it protects the human body from cold because it is a good isolator of heat therefore, we can notice that the lithe people feel cold weather more intensive that those who are obese because the obese individuals have a thicker protective layer of adipose tissue than the lithe individuals.

The obese people have higher weights than the lithe people. This is because of the adipose tissue that their body have. This high abnormal weight is considered a big load on the joints and the cartilage of the human body especially the knee joint which can cause pains in this region. Osteoarthritis is the inflammation of the joints and it may occur in some joints of the obese persons. It has been proved that adipose tissue in the stomach region increases the tendency of being sick in diabetes type II. Diabetes type II is a chronic disease that characterized by insufficient insulin stimulation to the muscle tissues that lead to insufficient entrance of glucose molecules to the muscle cells. This leads to the inability of muscle cells to function normally i.e. to contract.

An obese person has a higher risk to be affected by a high blood pressure. The normal blood pressure is 120/80 mm Hg. 120 mm Hg represents the systolic blood pressure and it is the blood pressure when the heart muscle contracts while 80 mm Hg is the diastolic blood pressure and it is the blood pressure when the heart muscle relaxes. The abnormal systolic blood pressure is higher than 140 mm Hg and the abnormal diastolic blood pressure is higher than 100 mm Hg.

Obese persons may have a high blood pressure because the heart muscle must pump the blood harder to reach all the cells of the human body which is bigger in size in obese persons. High blood pressure predisposes the person to a higher risk of stroke (the insufficient blood flow to the brain cells). Stroke because of overweight occurs because the arteries that nourish the brain regions burst or they become blocked.

LDL (low density lipoprotein or bad cholesterol) may be elevated in the blood of the obese persons. This high level of LDL predisposes to higher risk of atherosclerosis of the arteries.

Multivitamins and Minerals Supplements

The human body needs vitamins and minerals in little amounts in order to be alive. The main natural source of vitamins and minerals are fresh vegetables and fruits. They are essential for the biological reactions that occur in the human body. There are two types of vitamins depending on the ability of dissolving in water or lipids (fat) inside the human body. The lipid soluble vitamins are vitamins that are stored in the adipose tissue (fat tissue) of the human body. These are vitamins A, D, E and K. The water-soluble Vitamins are vitamins that are dissolved in water of the human body and they can not be stored inside the human body. The water-soluble vitamins are vitamin C and B.

Since fat soluble vitamins are stored inside the human body in the fat tissues, they can be toxic in high doses while water soluble vitamins which can not be stored inside the human body are not toxic in high doses.

The only source of high doses of vitamins are the multivitamin and minerals tablets or pills but not the fruit and vegetables which as said before, they the main natural sources of the vitamins and minerals.

Minerals, on the other side are many and they are also essential for the biological reactions inside the human body. The human body need the minerals in relatively higher amount than the vitamins. They are stored inside the human body and they also can be toxic in higher doses than normal.

The deficiency of each vitamin or mineral can predispose the human body for diseases. The toxicity and the diseases that are caused by the intake of abnormal doses of vitamins and minerals reflects the fact that the human body is a very precise and complicated biological system that functions in harmony and precision in relation to the diet that we eat. The human body will dysfunction if the doses of the vitamins and minerals will not be in the normal range.

From the evolutionary point of view, the human body has been adapted through millions of years to process the amounts of the vitamins and minerals that are existing naturally in the fruits and vegetables and other type of foods. Therefore, the varied diet is a better source of vitamins and minerals than the multivitamins and minerals pills that are found in the natural health stores. These multivitamins and minerals pills contain only few percent of the total number of the vitamins and minerals that the body need daily. Beside that, they do not contain certain compounds that are known as phytochemicals such as the substances that give the fruits and vegetables their characteristic colours. These phytochemicals are powerful antioxidants that are essential in fighting the free radicals that are produced by the body. The free radicals cause damages to the components of the cells including their DNA which if they proceed for a long period of time, they can cause many diseases in the human body including cancers. Therefore, the phytochemicals (and the vitamins and the minerals) are compounds that are very good in fighting cancer cells even before they arise in the human body.

Our biological system and its ability to process the food inside the human body is a unique reflection of our genes of our chromosomes. Our human genes have evolved through millions of years and because the genes are responsible for the manufacturing of the enzymes and all factors that are involved in every biological process, they (the genes) are responsible for all the biological processes inside the human body. Every biological reaction inside and outside the human cell is originated indeed from the human genes indirectly as explained before and therefore, the human genes are responsible for the metabolism inside the human body.

We can not change our genes depending upon the amount and or the type of the diet that we eat but we can change the type and or the amount of the diet that we eat in such way that is suitable for our pathways of metabolism. Consequently, the type of the food and or the amount of the specific diet that we eat should be suitable for the metabolic system of the human body. The metabolism is the process by which the food that we eat convert to the energy as ATP (Adenosine triphosphate) molecules. That type of metabolism is known as catabolism while the opposite type of metabolism is known as anabolism and it means that the body uses ATP molecule (energy molecule) to build up the components of the cells and the tissues such as the enzymes, the proteins, the lipids, the carbohydrates, etc. inside the human body.

The fact that few vitamins and minerals cannot cooperate for better health for the cells of the human body is essential in understanding the importance of the availability of all vitamins, minerals and phytochemicals that can be found in the fresh vegetables and fruits and other food. The totality of these vitamins and minerals that is founded naturally in each fresh fruit and vegetable boost and cooperate with each other in different biological reactions inside and outside the human cells. Therefore, eating fruits and vegetables are more beneficial than taking multivitamins and minerals pills. That rule is true in persons that do not have severe deficiency of certain vitamins and minerals or they need extra vitamins and minerals like the pregnant women.

Sleeping Rhythm

There is a variation in the rhythm of every day because the earth moves around itself. It completes a whole turn in 24 hours. The sunny hours and the dark hours during the nights. The whole earth moves around the sun and completes a whole turn in one year. The whole solar system moves in curvy way. Therefore, everything in the universe is in a continuous movement. There is a famous quote for the Greek philosopher Hermes Trismegistus that says: "As above as below" which means that the humans are nothing but a reflection of the whole unseen universe which is infinity in its dimensions if we see it from the traditional physical laws.

The sleeping rhythm is a mirror to the movement of the earth around itself that leads to the sunny day and the dark night periods of time.

Consequently, the human beings and almost all animals sleep during the nights and are awake during the day.

This rhythmic feature of wakefulness and sleep does have a reason that is very beneficial for the health of the human being. If we look at the EEG (Electro cardio gram) that measure the brain waves of different region inside the human brain we can see that during the sleep, these brain waves are different from the brain waves when the person is awake. The difference between the two patterns of the brain waves reveals that the conscious regions of the human brain that are alert when the person is awake, is in fact higher in amplitude compared to the brain waves that dominate during sleep which characterised by relatively low amplitudes. Although, during dreaming, there are some regions of the human brain that are relatively more active and have brain waves that are relatively high. These specific regions are responsible for the visual, memorial and emotional impulses inside the human brain.

There are two main types of sleep. The slow wave sleep and rapid eye movement sleep (REM). The former is a deep sleep and the body get more peaceful rest during it while the second is characterized by dreams that can be remembered and higher muscular tension and respiratory rate. The REM is occurred in 90 minutes interval during the whole night.

The physiological effect of the sleep is huge. It restores the balance and the rest to most of the brain regions from the higher intellectual regions like the cortex to the nonvoluntary activities of the human brain like the regions that regulate the blood pressure, muscular contraction and behavioural activities. The absence of sleep for a quite long time can cause exhaustion, irritability, aggressiveness and even psychotic behaviour. A hormone that is released from the pineal gland in the brain is known as melatonin and it is responsible for the rhythmic sleep pattern of the human being. The hormone begins to be released in the beginning of the evening and continue in high level in the blood stream until the sunrise in the morning. This hormone is essential for a good and deep sleep and there are many factors that influence its secretion such as the absence or presence of the day light, stress and trauma. It is better that you have your rum dark without any lamp turned on when you get to bed in order to allow the melatonin hormone to be secreted which in turn, allow the person to fall to sleep. There are many things that you can do to make your sleep deeper and better. You can for example jog at the evening for 30 minutes. That will release the natural endorphins into the blood stream that calm you down and make you relax. Jogging and physical exercise at the evening increase the blood flow to the pineal gland that is mentioned earlier which means that the pineal gland will function normally because of higher blood flow to its tissues. You can also drink a cup of worm milk since the milk have certain amino acid that enhance sleep.

You can listen to a calm music before bed time which relax you and make you to fall to sleep. You should avoid coffee at least five hours before bed time because the caffeine in the coffee is a very powerful stimulant for the central nervous system (the brain and the spinal cord) and it inhibits the mechanism that initiates the sleep in the human being.

Water Drinking

The water constitutes most of the mass of the human body. Almost every tissue inside the human body contains water molecules. Without water the human body can not survive. The water molecules participate in every biological reaction inside and outside the human cells.

From the evolutionary point of view, water is considered the origin of life on earth. There are many researches that have proved that the origin of life started in the water of oceans and the water of floods as primitive microorganism that had had the ability of movement inside the water. Through millions of years of evolution of the human being, the life had transmitted from the water to the beaches and gradually to the forests where the human being in its existing form had lived.

The water was the fundamental factor in the evolution of all animal kingdom, including the human beings.

If we look at the animal kingdoms and all its races, we can see that all the living creatures drink water in order to survive.

The water molecule is one of the simplest molecules that can be found. It is composed of two hydrogen atoms and one oxygen atoms. The chemical bound between the hydrogen and the oxygen atom is covalent. The water molecule has a low molecular weight, but it has a very beneficial effect on all the biological reactions inside the human body.

The most characteristic feature of the water from the biological point of view is that it can be secreted in various amount with urine. The urine contains almost water molecules.

The detoxification of the toxins, medical molecules and alcohol for examples occur in the liver. The liver has many functions in the human body and one of the most important function is to detoxify the blood from the waste products. The blood reflects for a certain degree, the purity of the surrounding tissues and cells. Therefore, every toxic molecule that can be found in the tissues and the cells, it could be found in the surrounding blood flow. The blood transport nutrients and oxygen to the cells and it also transport the waste products and carbon dioxide from the cells. Almost all those waste products are secreted outside the human body through the urine.

But what is the role of water in all of that? Well, the water that we drink is transported to the blood through the absorption from the intestine, especially, the colon. When we drink a moderate and enough water daily, we dilute the blood since the water is absorbed through the colon into the blood stream as said before. This dilution of the blood decreases the osmolarity of the blood and increase the blood total volume. Consequently, the blood must get rid of this excessive amount of water in the blood through the urination process in order to maintain the osmolarity and the volume of the blood in the normal range which is very important for the physiology of the blood.

Because the urination is one of the biological processes by which the human body can get rid of waste products and toxic substances outside the human body, the water that we drink is a key factor in the frequency by which we urinate daily. i.e. whenever a high amount is drunk daily there is a high amount of secreted urine outside the human body. That means, there is a higher amount of waste products and toxic substances being secreted through the urine. The conclusion is that whenever we drink a high amount of water, we get rid of a higher amount of waste products and toxic substances.

If we drink high amount of coffee, there will be retention of waste products and toxic substances inside the human body since the coffee stimulate the urination even when there is a small amount of urine in the bladder. Therefore, under periods of heavy coffee drinking, we should drink higher amount of water.

Meditation

There is a reciprocal relationship between the physical human body and the psychological condition of the human being. Meditation achieved in the human physical body and the human psychological condition when the person try to make the body receives many stimuli through the physical human body and through his five senses.

There are many types of meditation and they are quite various and diverse in their methods, procedures and results.

Yoga for example, focuses on many bodily postures that the one can do to achieve a certain result in feelings and the physical human strength and endurance.

The more we learn about meditation and practicing what we learn, the more we get a better result. The patience in this issue is very important. It could take many years to get a complete benefit of each exercise in meditation.

Our five senses are very important in the meditation's exercise. These five senses include: the smell, the touch, the vision, the hearing and the taste senses.

When we incorporate these five senses or some of them into our meditation sessions, we increase the benefit we get from each exercise of meditation.

Most of the meditation's sessions are achieved with closed eyes because opened eye will disturb the concentration and the focus on what we want to concentrate on.

The visualization of many views during meditation is essential in many types of meditation. The vision is a very sensitive and accurate sense that the human body has during his life. When we use this tool i.e. the visualization of certain scenarios with a closed eye, we make our emotions resonate with the visual scenario that is chosen. When we change our emotions in this way, we manipulate our aura because the changing in the aura is affected by the change of our emotions and vice versa. Many things about the aura is discussed in detail in the following book: The Unknown about the Human Aura – The Human Aura from a Medical Point of View.

When the aura (the astral field) changes in dimensions and colours intensities, the emotions of the person will change at the same time.

When we meditate, we usually focus our attention on an object, colour, an ide or a scenario of moving pictures. The only thing that characterized all those methods of thinking is that they are all positive for the health in an indirect way.

If we think about a specific colour for example, it should be a light colour instead of thinking about a dark colour. You should avoid thinking of or visualizing the black colour and all its grades of intensities because it is very harmful for the human aura and consequently it is very harmful for the human physical body and the health in general.

Each colour you think about will be reflected in your aura and gradually your aura will be transformed to a bright shiny aura after many sessions of meditation with colour visualization. If your aura (the biological fields that surrounds the human body) becomes healthier (brighter) then, it reflects itself in the physical human body and the human body becomes more healthier and purer.

When a person thinks about specific objects like a flower or a river, etc. the person will have peaceful feeling and calmness in the mind and the sole. This is true for every technique that the person practices in meditation session. Beside that, the person will have a better sleep pattern and its anxiety level will be decreased. The hormone serotonin is secreted during the meditation and the natural endorphins and enkephalins. Therefore, the person feels calmness and happiness after each meditation session. The person will show an increased tolerance for different stressful situations in daily life. A specific mantra can be accompanied during meditation. The mantras are different sounds that can be pronounced or listened during meditation. It is very helpful in calming down the human body and remove any tensions that could be found in the human body.

Acupuncture

Acupuncture is an old therapeutic Chinese method that is used until today to heal many health problems. It uses small needles that are inserted few millimetres inside the skin of the patient. These needles are distributed in certain way over the skin according to the type of the health problem that the patient suffers from.

The patient should be relaxed during acupuncture session. The mechanism of action of these needles is not known for many people yet. These needles are made of metal and they are flexible at the same time. They are inserted in the skin in positions that are related to the meridians of the human body. The meridians are lines that the qi or the vital energy passes through after they are entering through the chakra system of the human body. There are seven chakras and they are located in the midline of the human body. These chakras are classified as following: the seventh chakra is the crown chakra that are situated at the top of the head and its colour is violet. The sixth chakra is the ajna chakra or the third eye chakra which is situated at the forehead between the eyebrows and its colour is purple. The fifth chakra is the throat chakra which is situated at the neck region and its colour is blue. The fourth chakra is the heart chakra and it is situated at the horizontal line of the heart region and its colour is green. The third chakra is solar plexus chakra and it is situated at the navel and its colour is yellow. The second chakra is the sacral chakra and it is located at the lumbar region of the vertebral column and its colour is orange. The first chakra is the base chakra and it is situated at the end of the vertebral column and its colour is red.

Those chakras receive the cosmic energy or the vital force from the universe and distribute it throughout the whole human body through the meridian lines as mentioned earlier.

The flow of the vital force from the cosmos into the meridians that are spread throughout the human body, with the help of the seven chakras, seizes after the death of the human body. Therefore, that force is known as the vital force because it supplies the human body with the healing power and the power of life that the one needs in order to survive.

There is a period when the clinical symptoms of the disease are not manifested in the human body. This period usually before the period of the clinical symptoms which are obvious and can be measured or seen by the traditional medicine.

The first period of "subclinical" symptoms is what the Chinese medicine deal with by the acupuncture and the Chinese herbs. If the patient does not heal himself with the Chinese medicine in the first period then, the therapy of the second period when the symptoms become clinical, becomes more difficult.

The acupuncture needles modulate the flow of the vital energy or the Qi energy through the human body in such way that the equilibrium of the vital energy is restored. Most of the health problems inside the human body begins with imbalance in the vital energy flow among the chakras and the vital energy flow among different organs of the human body.

Massage

The massage and its various types has been existing in the human history since ancient times. The main principle of massage is based on the physical touching that is applied on the skin of the human body by the pressure of touching of the fingers, palms, elbows and feet.

The pressure on the skin of the human body stimulates the mechanoreceptors that are situated inside the layers of the skin. Those mechanoreceptors are connected by nerve fibres to the central nervous system (the brain and the spinal cord). Therefore, the touching stimulates the release of serotonin and endorphins from the central nervous system into the blood stream. Those substances induce the feelings of happiness, joyfulness and relaxation. They relieve neurological tension and relaxes skeletal muscles of the human body.

They also decrease the depression's symptoms and give euphoria feelings for the person. They are essentials in decreasing the physical pain that can be existing in some parts of the human body.

There are many other ways to achieve those aims of the massage beside the physical touching of the human body. These ways include scents, vapoured water, calming music, etc.

Oil, cream or lotions are usually used during massage session in order to decrease the friction between the hands and the skin of the human body.

There are four main types of mechanoreceptors (sensory receptors) and they are either classified according to the size of the sensory field on the surface of the skin or the speed by which the nerve fibres that are connected to the mechanoreceptors, transmit the nerve impulses to the central nervous system.

All the four mechanoreceptors in the skin are sensitive to pressure or distortion of the skin tissue. These mechanoreceptors are connected to nerve fibres that transmit the nerve impulses which are originated when the mechanoreceptors become stimulated by pressure or distortion of the skin. The nerve fibres transmit the nerve impulses to a region inside the human brain which is known as the thalamus. From the thalamus another nerve fibres transmit the nerve impulses to another important region of the human brain which is known as the cerebral sensory cortex. The cerebral sensory cortex enables us to feel the different objects that touch our skin.

The main hormone which is secreted in the blood stream during the tactile pressure of massage is called oxytocin. Oxytocin is synthesized from the hypothalamus of the brain and transmitted to the posterior lobe of the pituitary gland which is situated at the base of the brain. Oxytocin is secreted from the pituitary gland to the blood stream and binds to its receptors on different cell types in the human body.

After binding to its receptors that are situated on the cells, its effects begin to appear in the tissue and the organ. Oxytocin has receptors in the brain tissues, the cells of the smooth muscles and the breast glands. Oxytocin is a polypeptide hormone that has many functions and positive effects on both the human body and the psychological condition of the human beings. Oxytocin makes the person feels good and satisfied. It increases the libido (the desire of sex).

The oxytocin has also receptors on the skeletal muscles and therefore, the increased level of the oxytocin in the blood stream by massage and other stimuli, increases the numbers of the skeletal muscles.

Oxytocin have a halve time of about three minutes in the blood. Therefore, we can notice that whenever the massage stimuli are ceased, the effects of the oxytocin in the human body is ceased too.